Pharmacy Technician Certification Study Guide

Key Points Exam Prep Team

Pharmacy Technician Certification Study Guide:

Copyright © 2015 Key Points Exam Prep Team

All rights reserved. No part of this book may be reproduced or transmitted in any form or by any means without written permission from the author.

ISBN-13: 978-1505729351

ISBN-10: 1505729351

Printed in the United States of America.

Table of Contents

Regulations and Technical Duties

Overview of Technician's Duties

General Information

The Role of the Pharmacist and the Pharmacy Technician

What a Pharmacy Technician May NOT Do

Prescription Department Layout and Workflow

Pharmacy Security

Inventory Control

Stocking Medications

Identifying Expired Products

Controlled Substances

Difference among Controlled Substances Schedules

Refills, partial refills, filing, and prescription transfers

Correct procedures for handling Schedule V sales

Controlled Substance Act

DEA numbers

Other Laws and Regulation

Federal Privacy Act

Generic Substitution

Professionals with Prescribing Authority

Regulations and Technical Duties

In order for a pharmacy technician to be registered or certified that person must be a member of the College of Pharmacists. Since membership varies from country to country and American state to state, it is wise to research the regulations for the state in which you will be licensed and working. There is no universal rule governing the licensing of pharmaceutical technicians throughout United States. However many American states and provinces have their own regulations regarding certification.

In some states regulation is voluntary. However, being unlicensed has some drawbacks in job opportunities, responsibilities, and remuneration.

The regulation holds a pharmacy technician responsible, accountable and liable for a his/her specific duties. Those specific duties will be discussed in detail in a later section.

Overview of Technician's Duties

An overview of the job of the pharmacy technician includes such duties as: working under the supervision of a pharmacist to assist in providing medication and health care products to clients. Technicians' routine tasks often include preparing prescribed medication like as counting tablets and labeling bottles.

General Information

The pharmacy technician supports pharmacological services in a store or department by stocking inventory, assembling medications as directed by the pharmacist, and distributing medications.

The qualified pharmacy technician has no uniform specific certification until 2020. In the United States, there is as yet no regulatory agency governing the training of Pharmacy Technicians. Every state has a Board of Pharmacy which is in charge of licensing Pharmacy Technicians.

Moreover, requirements vary widely with some states requiring training from a board-approved school, PTCB certification, and/or a period of apprenticeship. Some states have no requirements.

In addition to whatever formal training is required, pharmacy technicians need to possess the following skills and abilities:

- Understanding and execution of supply management
- Organizational skills
- Integrity and a sense of confidentiality
- Strong reporting skills
- Keen attention to detail
- Dependability, honesty
- Ability to create a safe, effective working environment
- Focus on quality
- Analytical, able to analyze information
- Effective communication skills

The Role of the Pharmacist and the Pharmacy Technician

A licensed pharmacist performs the following duties:

1. **Dispense Prescription Medications**

    Pharmacists count tablets, prepare bottle label and handle medications to patients.

2. **Interact with Prescribing Physicians**

    If a prescription order is unclear or potentially harmful for a patient, the pharmacist confirms the dosage and medicine form, as well as whether brand name or a generic product may be substituted.

3. **Ensure Customer Safety**

   Each time a client gets a prescription or a refill, the pharmacist checks the client's medication record to ensure the prescription will not create a dangerous reaction with his/her other medications.

4. **Dialogue with Customers**

   The pharmacist warns his customers of any potentially adverse reactions between his other medications and/or food, beverages, or alcohol. The pharmacist also listens to patient concerns and makes suggestions regarding when medication should be taken or if the patient should be making an appointment to discuss adverse reactions with his doctor.

5. **Discuss General Health Concerns**

   Pharmacists can help patients improve or maintain their general health by providing suggestions regarding over-the-counter products, health supplements herbal remedies, diet, and/or exercise.

6. **Work with Insurance Companies and Government Plans**

   Pharmacists are required to have knowledge of insurance claims, work with insurance companies and submit claims forms. They often work with clients to resolve denied insurance claims.

7. **Manage Staff**

   Pharmacists must work with, mentor, and supervise staff including pharmacy technicians to ensure that each client receives the right drug in the correct dose.

8. **Organize and Secure Patient Records**

   Whether the job is done by a pharmacy technician or the pharmacist himself, pharmacists are responsible for the correct maintenance, accuracy, and security of each client file.

9. **Keep Medical Personnel Apprised of New Drugs**

   Because he works with drugs, the pharmacist must be current on new drugs and keep physicians and other medical staff with whom he deals up to date on the newest drugs.

   The pharmaceutical technician has the following responsibilities:

   - Assist health care providers and patients by answering questions and requests, referring inquiries to the pharmacist.
   - Maintain the pharmacy stock by checking to determine inventory level
   - The pharmacy technician anticipates required medications and supplies, places and expedites orders
   - The pharmacy technician verifies receipt of new supplies, removes and replaces outdated drugs.
   - The pharmacy technician is responsible for maintaining a safe, clean pharmacy.
   - The pharmacy technician knows, and complies with all pharmacy procedures, rules, and regulations.

- The pharmacy technician adheres to infection-control policies and protocols so patients and pharmacy staff are protected against infections and diseases.

- The pharmacy technician organizes medications so the pharmacist can dispense medications and prescriptions easily.

- The pharmacy technician reads prescriptions, prepares labels, calculate quantities, assembles intravenous solutions and other pharmaceutical supplies under the supervision of the pharmacist.

- The pharmacy technician files physicians' orders and prescriptions, maintaining patient files.

- The pharmacy technician calculates fees, records charges, and issues bills.

- If working in a medical facility, the pharmacy technician delivers medications to patients and/or departments.

- The pharmacy technician collects and summarizing information for reports.

- Operating as part of a pharmacy team, the pharmacy technician completed requested tasks required by the pharmacist.

What a Pharmacy Technician May NOT Do

- Pharmacy technicians may NOT fill prescriptions. They can assist the pharmacy by putting labels on the bottles or recording prescription information in the patient's file.

- Pharmacy technicians may NOT assess appropriateness of a prescription drug.

- Pharmacy technician do not dialogue with medical professionals regarding potential adverse effects of prescribed medications.

- Pharmacy technician do not discuss with clients cautions regarding possible interaction of drugs, food, beverages and/or alcohol.

- Pharmacy technicians do not keep medical personnel apprised of new drugs.

- Pharmacy technicians do not interact with insurance companies, file claims, or attempt to resolve issues with denied drug claims.
- Pharmacy technicians do not counsel patients on clinical issues although they may discuss healthy habits such as diet or exercise.

Prescription Department Layout and Workflow

Because orders come from a variety of sources and in various paths, a pharmacy's work space must be set up to receive prescriptions in person, by phone and fax and via the Internet. Most prescriptions will arrive with the patient in the form of a paper copy prescription from his doctor. However, getting new and repeat prescriptions in the form of phone, fax, or Internet is becoming increasingly common.

To avoid confusion there should be clearly designated work stations for each staff member, an in window to receive prescriptions and an out window to dispense prescriptions and a data entry area. The medications area should have clearly labeled and organized shelves, bins, bottles to be filled, and locked cabinets for narcotics.

If the order is an existing or new prescription the pharmacist or pharmacy technician first checks patients files for any allergies or other medications that might interact negatively with this prescription. As other medications or health conditions may have changed it is necessary to check for potential problems each time. Finding none, the prescription is filled. Cautions and directions for taking the medication are attached to the package. Medical quick orders are filled out for future refills indicating: renew; discontinue; copy to new order; change medication. Orders are then signed and the prescription filled in store, by e-prescription to another pharmacy, or to another department in the facility.

Patients and doctors can phone in refills using Automated Voice Response (AVR). When a patient phones in a request for a refill or a doctor calls in a new or repeat prescription, the same steps are taken to ensure no allergies or conflicts in medication. Forms and record keeping follows the same procedure and the prescription is prepared for patient pick up or delivery.

Regardless of how many or few prescriptions are filled each day, the pharmacy's prescription department must be set up for maximum efficiency. This means the path to filling the individual prescription must be set up so personnel are not getting in each other's way and they are required to take as few steps as possible. While computerization of patient records, and printing of labels has greatly eased the workflow, there is still the potential for poor organization of traffic spaces.

Another thing to consider is division of labor. Whose job is it to receive prescriptions by hard copy, phone, fax, and computer? Who checks patients' medical records to ensure safety? Are these checks initialed by the pharmacist? Who fills the prescription? Does this vary depending on the type of medication? Who prints the labels? Who interacts with the patient going over cautions? Who is responsible for record keeping of patient's file and for billing? Is there a second person check on these files?

The answers to the above questions will vary from pharmacy to pharmacy but they should be consistent within that facility so there are no misunderstandings or omissions. The facility should operate like a well-oiled machine. Work should flow smoothly and the physical plant should be set up so that everything is up to date. All staff know where everything is and someone—often the pharmacy technician—is responsible for taking inventory, reordering and restocking shelves.

Pharmacy Security

Because pharmacies deal with sought-after drugs it is necessary to have multiple and state-of-the-art security. While security is not the responsibility of the pharmacy technician, it is important that the pharmacy assistant know the security systems that are in place and how to operate them. It is also advisable that the pharmacy technician suggest areas that are not properly secured to his/her immediate superior. These areas must be considered.

a) **Alarms**
   Does the system have an alarm system?
   Is there battery backup in case of a power outage?
   Is this a silent or audible alarm? Is there a flashing light visual alarm?
   Where is the alarm button?
   What checks exist in case of a false alarm?
   Is the alarm system supervised or unsupervised?
   What areas are alarmed: doors, windows, roof entrances, high security areas?
   Are the adjoining business walls alarmed?

b) **Keys**
   Limited issuance?
   Do not duplicate protected?
   Numbered keys?
   Opening and Closing procedures in place?

c) **Sensors**
   Motion detectors
   Trap alarm
   Glass breaking
   Fire
   Duress
   Vibration

d) **Physical Barriers**
   Steel window and/or door curtains?
   Pharmacy department doors?
   Barriers to prevent jumping into the dispensing area?
   Bollards outside the pharmacy?
   Interior safe?

e) **Closed Circuit TV**
   At all entrance doors?
   On parking lot?
   Drive through window camera?
   Hidden camera at customer counters- face level view?

Regular weekly audit and maintenance of cameras and recorded materials?
Hidden, secured recorder?

f) **Camera**
Digital?
Black and white or color?
Variable focus lens?
Low level light capabilities?

g) **Recordings**
Archived?
Retained?
Digital?
Tapes/disks replaced regularly?
Ten + frames per second?

h) **Burglary**
Policy and procedures clearly developed, in place, and rehearsed?
Police involved in staff training and rehearsal?
911 Emergency and alarm directly to police?
Know procedures in case of break in to protect evidence?
Details of crime forms in place?
Keep surfaces clean so that fingerprints and other forensic evidence is easy to obtain?
Police response time?

i) **Process for**
Ordering?
Delivering?
Accepting returns?
Drug bottles identified with pharmacy ID?

Inventory Control

Accurate inventory control is important in any business. In the pharmacy business it is even more critical because people's health is at stake. Your training as a pharmacy technician your training will have included an appreciate for the importance of making sure all medical stock—whether in a commercial or institutional setting—is current so you are able to fill orders the moment they are needed. Many times, prescriptions are needed immediately. Successfully dispensing prescriptions must be done efficiently and the inventory organized and readily available.

Good inventory control ensures that patients get their medication at the lowest cost. Inventory costs may vary from season to season and year to year as well as company to company. Controlling the inventory of your pharmacy aims to:

- Minimize the cost of overstocking and having to discard out-of-date medications
- Maintain sufficient stock so the patient always has his needed prescription in a timely manner.
- Minimize the cost of overstocks and small emergency orders.
- Knowing exactly what is in stock at any given time.

Inventory control in a pharmacy enterprise is often difficult because of changing medications of existing clients, walk in clients, changing demographics of the business area. Often inventory control is one of the duties assigned to a pharmacy technician. Pharmacies are expected to keep a wide variety of stock. They are also expected to turn over their inventory without extra costs of out-of-date medications whose cost must be passed on to the customer. They are expected to make bulk purchases to save money while balancing that against overstock costs.

Inventory Control Methods

a) The "open-to-buy budget" method allots funds in a specific timeframe, to buy pharmaceutical inventory.
b) The "short-list" method singles of products in low stock and flags these for the pharmaceutical technician to replace.
c) The "minimum and maximum" method seeks to discover how much of each item to order and the best time financially to order those items.
d) Like library stock, the "stock card" method traces when items are purchased by using notations on cards or e-cards.

Stocking Medications

While stocking inventory is important to any business it can well be a life-and-death issue in a pharmacy setting. Medication errors are a shocking cause deaths in North America. Dispensing errors account for over 20% of medication mistakes. Besides the potential for loss of life, dispensing errors increase cost society in increased healthcare costs. Dispensing errors can also be a major economic liability to a pharmacy if the client decides to sue.

Dispensing errors are catastrophic for the client, his family, his doctor, and the pharmacy. Many dispensing errors can be eliminated if inventory is stored in carefully marked, consistent locations so everyone involved in filling prescriptions automatically knows where every medication is located.

As the professional responsible for restocking shelves, the pharmacy technician must ensure medications are clearly marked and the organization is logical. Organizing work space, work environment, and workflow significantly reduces dispensing errors. Ensure good lighting, clear counter space, and optimum temperature and humidity facilitates work flow, reducing the chances of dispensing errors. Another good strategy in stocking medications is to deal with one medication at a time including dispensing and labeling the medication with the patient's name, medication, dosage, and additional instructions. This will help prevent medication mix-ups. Never leave any drug containers unlabeled.

Mix-ups also occur more readily when drugs look alike. To avoid grabbing the wrong one, store them away from each other in the medication storage area. Medication bottles should be properly organized with labels facing front where they can easily be read.

Identifying Expired Products

It can be dangerous to use out-of-date drugs. Not to mention it is unethical and illegal for pharmacies to sell past date products. Pharmacy technicians should routinely check all medications on the shelves. Expired medications should be discarded. Use of storage bins, cabinets, or drawers can result in misplacement of look-alike drugs. It is also advisable to lock up or sequester drugs with high potential of causing errors.

The process of taking expired medications off the shelves is complicated by the fact that expiry dates can vary dramatically. For example: expiry in injectable epinephrine "Epipens" is notoriously unstable. Most injectable epinephrine product expires 18 months after the product arrives for stocking on the shelves. Other drug products must be stored in special containers because they are highly sensitive to moisture. Many liquid antibiotics are unstable and must, thus, be prepared at the time they are dispensed. Many drugs—including vaccine and eye drops—require or they will become unstable and must then be discarded.

Pharmacy technicians who are often responsible for discarding drugs that are past their expiry date should be aware that the expiry date is based on testing of unopened products, stored in their original container, and maintained exactly as specified.

Opening bottles or packages or transferring drugs to another container makes the manufacturer's expiry date no longer valid. The stability of the medication may be compromised if it is introduced to light, heat, or humidity.

Many drug companies provide specific "use by" and "do not use after" labels to guide the expiry date process of discarding drugs. Some even provide a program whereby expired drugs can be returned to the manufacturer for safe disposal and a rebate for replacing the expired drugs with current ones.

Pharmaceutical technicians also need to be aware of regulations regarding the safe disposal of expired drugs for their jurisdiction. Depending on the form of medication and the regulations of the area it could be as simple as trash discard, packaging for return to manufacturer or disposal as a hazardous waste at a specific site and time.

Record keeping of what drugs, in what quantities, where, when and how the drug was disposed of are vital for regulations as well as for pharmacy accounting and inventory control. The pharmacy needs to have in place a clear procedure for dealing with expired medications. The procedure must be set in place, monitored and the destruction witnessed by a licensed pharmacist.

Controlled Substances

Safeguarding controlled substances is a concern for manufacturers, distributors, and pharmacies. Federal law specifies that handling of controlled substances requires their proper safeguarding at all times. The drug Enforcement Administration (DEA) is in charge ensuring that proper security is maintained.

Safe storage and sales of controlled substances are regulated by such federal laws as Controlled Drugs and Substances Act, Narcotics Control Regulations, and Food and Drug Administration Regulations.

Any controlled drug is a substance set out in Food and Drug Regulations, Part G. All controlled substances in North America must have an eight-digit DIN numerical code in accordance with the Food and Drugs Act and Food and Drug Regulations to be sold legally. This includes drugs intended for human and veterinary purposes.

Moreover, there are specific regulations regarding the safe handling, storage, and dispensing of controlled substances. Handlers of controlled substances need to be alert to diversion methods regarding controlled substances. These include illegal sale, falsified prescription orders, burglary, employee theft, loss in-transit, robbery, and patient theft.

An important step in preventing the diversion of controlled substances is employee screening. Anyone working in a pharmacy is in a position to have contract with controlled substances. Employees should be screened before they are hired to identify potential security problems. This should include evaluation of the applicant's personal and previous employment references as well as criminal background checks with local law enforcement and DEA. The same caution should be taken when employees are transferred to new jobs where controlled substances exist.

Areas to be protected against theft and diversion of controlled substances vary greatly depending on the individual pharmacy. All controlled substances areas must be secured. The pharmacist must secure both the controlled substance storage and prescription dispensing areas. The number of employees who work in these areas must be limited and access controlled and monitored.

Factors to consider in securing controlled substances must include:

- Activity conducted in handling controlled substances such as: processing of bulk chemicals, preparing dosage forms, packaging, labelling, and dispensing of the controlled substance.
- Form of controlled substances including: bulk liquids, dosage units, usable powders or non-usable powders.
- Quantity of controlled substances in the pharmacy.
- Location of the business regarding security needs. Is the pharmacy located in a high or low crime area? Is waterfront located near the building? Are there any adjacent or attached buildings? Is the pharmacy in an urban, suburban or rural area?
- What type of building construction is the pharmacy? Is the structure: metal curtain, wood frame or masonry? How many doors, windows and other openings does the building have? What is the material of doors? Are there safes, vaults, and/or other secure enclosures including: automatic storage and retrieval? Of what material are vaults and cages constructed? What is the GSA rating of security systems. How are security areas opened and closed? Are there built-in combination locks, key locks, padlocks, self-closing and locking day gates? How are entrance and exit to controlled substance areas monitored? Is the alarm system adequately supervised? How are burglary or intrusions signaled? How is public access to the building and the property supervised and controlled.
- Who monitors employee movement? How is employee access to the controlled substances area(s) monitored?

Difference among Controlled Substances Schedules

What are Controlled Substances Schedules?

Drugs and medications considered controlled substances under the Controlled Substances Act (CSA) are divided into five schedules. These are outlined in the annual *Title 21 Code of Federal Regulations (C.F.R.) §§ 1308.11 through 1308.15.* The designation of schedules is based on whether the controlled substance currently has an FDA approved medical use in treatment in the United States. The designation also considers the relative abuse potential of each controlled substance, and the likelihood of that substance's causing dependence if it is abused.

Schedule I

Substances with no currently accepted medical use. These substances lack accepted safety for medical use and have a high potential for abuse.

Examples: heroin, lysergic acid diethylamide (LSD), marijuana (cannabis), peyote, methaqualone, and methylenedioxymethamphetamine (Ecstasy).

Schedule II

These controlled substances have a high potential for abuse. This abuse could lead to severe psychological or physical dependence.

Examples: Examples of Schedule II narcotics include: hydromorphone, methadone, Demerol, oxycodone, OxyContin, Percocet, and fentanyl, morphine, opium, codeine, and hydrocodone.

Schedule III:

Schedule Three substances have less potential for abuse than substances in Schedules One and Two. Abuse of Schedule Three substances may lead to moderate to low physical dependence or high psychological dependence.

Examples: Tylenol with Codeine, benzphetamine, phendimetrazine, ketamine, and anabolic steroids.

Schedule IV:

Schedule Four controlled substances have less potential for abuse than Schedule Three substances.

Examples: Xanax, Soma, Klonopin, Tranxene, Valium, Ativan, Versed, Restoril, and Halcion.

Schedule V:

These substances have the lowest potential for abuse of all controlled substances. They are mainly preparations containing limited quantities of certain narcotics.

Examples: cough syrups with less than 200 mg of codeine/100 ml such as Robitussin AC, Phenergan with Codeine, and Ezogabine.

Refills, partial refills, filing, and prescription transfers

A prescription must be dated and signed on the date it was issued. It must include: patient's full name and address, and the medical practitioner's full name, address, and his/her DEA registration number.

Included on the prescription must be:

- Name of the medication
- Strength
- Dosage form
- Quantity prescribed
- Directions for use
- Number of authorized refills—if any.

The prescription must be written in ink, indelible pencil or typewritten. It must be signed by the practitioner on the date of issue. A secretary or nurse may prepare prescriptions for the practitioner's signature. The practitioner is responsible for ensuring the prescription conforms to federal and state laws and regulations before he signs it.

Since March, 2010, electronic prescriptions have been allowed if they are prepared on accepted software. Only those electronic pharmacy applications that comply with all of DEA's requirements may be used and only by DEA-registered pharmacies permitted to receive and archive electronic prescriptions for controlled substances prescriptions and dispense controlled substances based on electronic prescriptions.

The pharmacy must use a pharmacy application that meets requirements of **21 C.F.R. §1311**.

The prescription conforms to the requirements of the CSA and **21 C.F.R. §1311**.

A pharmacy cannot refill a controlled substance. The refilling of a prescription for a controlled substance listed in schedule II is prohibited under regulation **21 U.S.C. § 829**(a)).

The DEA has revised regulations for multiple prescriptions for a Schedule II controlled substance. As of December 19, 2007, a doctor may issue multiple prescriptions for up to a ninety-day supply of Schedule II controlled substances as long as:

- Each prescription is on a separate prescription blank.
- Each prescription is for a medically legitimate purpose.
- The issuing physician has provided clear instructions re: the date each individual prescription may be filled.
- The physician issuing multiple prescriptions is confident multiple prescriptions are not part of drug abuse.
- Issuing multiple prescriptions is legal under state law.

- The issuing practitioner has complied with all requirements under the CSA and C.F.R., and any additional requirements under state law.

Schedules III and IV controlled substances <u>may</u> be refilled if a refill note was included on the prescription. Prescriptions may be refilled up to five times within six months after the date of issue. Beyond either five refills or after six month, a new prescription must be obtained.

Partial Filling

A pharmacist may partially fill a prescription for a schedule II controlled substance if the pharmacist cannot supply the full quantity of a written prescription or one which the physician phoned in in case of emergency. However, in the case of partial filling of a prescription, the pharmacist must make note of the quantity supplied on the written prescription, or on a written record of the emergency phone prescription, or on the electronic prescription record. The remaining prescription dose may be dispensed within three days of the partial filling. In the event that the remainder of the prescription cannot be filled in seventy-two hours, the pharmacist must notify the issuing doctor and a new prescription will be issued to replace the partially filled one.

A prescription for a schedule II substance of a patient in a Long Term Care Facility or one who is terminally illness, may be filled in partially filled. Both the pharmacist and the issuing doctor must be sure the prescription is indeed for that patient.

Correct procedures for handling Schedule V sales

Drugs classified in Schedule V of the Uniform Controlled Substances Act (RCW 69.50.212) can be dispensed without a prescription. However, the pharmacy selling Schedule V controlled substances must be confident that these products are being bought for medical intent as outlined on the manufacturer's label. Examples include cough syrups with small amounts of codeine.

Schedule V controlled substances can be sold under the following guidelines:

- The product is sold only by a licensed pharmacist, a pharmacy technician or a pharmacy intern.
- The pharmacist, pharmacy technician or pharmacy intern must recording of the information in the Schedule V register book.
- The pharmacist, pharmacy technician, or pharmacy intern may not sell a Schedule V drug to anyone under 21.
- The purchaser must supply identification to verify name, address and age.
- Schedule V drugs must be safeguarded in a locaton inaccessible to public.
- Name and address of the pharmacy selling the controlled substance must be affixed to the bottle or vial as well as the date of sale and the seller's initials.
- Every purchaser of a Schedule V product must be provided with a copy of subsections (3) and (4) of Schedule V drugs.
- Every pharmacy handling Schedule V drugs must have a Schedule V register book. At the top of each page should be the statement: "I have not obtained any Schedule V preparations within the last ninety-six hours, nor obtained Schedule V preparations more than twice within the last sixty days. This is my true name and address."
- All sales of Schedule V preparations without a doctor's prescription must be recorded in the Schedule V register including buyer's name, address, DOB, proof of identification, date of sale, name and quantity of controlled substance, initials of dispensing pharmacist, pharmacy technician or pharmacy intern an signature of the buyer.
- The register must be bound, 8 ½ x 11" book. All pages must be numbered. There must be an original and a duplicate of each page. The duplicate pages must be mailed to the pharmacy board at the end of each month.
- Registers must be available on request to the state pharmacy board of investigation.

Controlled Substance Act (CSA)

The Controlled Substances Act is an American federal policy that regulates manufacture, importing, possession, use and distribution of all substances deemed to be controlled as outlined by the CSA. It is known as Title II of the Comprehensive Drug Abuse Prevention and Control Act of 1970. The CSA is a vehicle for nation-wide implementing for the Single Convention on Narcotic Drugs.

The CSA created the schedule or classifications), with varying qualification of controlled substances into five schedules. The Drug Enforcement Administration (DEA) and the Food and Drug Administration (FDA) work together to decide what substances should be added, moved, or removed from each of the schedules.

A copy of the legislation is available at http://www.fda.gov/regulatoryinformation/legislation/ucm148726.htm

DEA Numbers

DEA registration numbers are assigned to a health care provider (for example: a doctor, dentist, or veterinarian. The American Drug Enforcement Administration thereby allows licensed healthcare providers to write prescriptions for controlled substances as outlined in Schedules I through V in the Controlled Substances Act. DEA numbers are used to track controlled substances.

The medical community also uses it as an identifier of prescription issuers. No one without a DEA number can prescribe medication in USA.

DEA numbers are comprised of two letters, six numbers and a check digit.

Other Laws and Regulation

In the United States, food, drugs, cosmetics, and medical devices are regulated by the Food and Drug Administration (FDA). The FDA regulations were created in response to concerns for public safety regarding food and medications. Created in 1931, the FDA a branch of the US Department of Health and Human Services (HHS). Other branches include: Centers for Disease Control and Prevention (CDC), National Institutes of Health (NIH), and Healthcare Financing Administration (HCFA).

The FDA is a law enforcement agency tasked with safeguarding. The FDA is not the only agency within the US government with a stake in pharmaceutical issues. The Federal Trade Commission (FTC) has authority over general business practices in general.

The FDA licenses and inspects manufacturing facilities. It tests products; evaluates claims and prescription drug advertising. The FDA also monitors research. It creates regulations, guidelines, standards, and policies through its Office of Operations. Component offices include: Center for Drug Evaluation and Research (CDER), the Center for Biologics Evaluation and Research (CBER), the Center for Devices and Radiological Health (CDRH), the Center for Food Safety and Applied Nutrition (CFSAN), the Center for Veterinary Medicine (CVM), the Office of Orphan Products Development, the Office of Biotechnology, the Office of Regulatory Affairs, and the National Center for Toxicological Research.

Most prescription drugs are evaluated by the CDER. The FDA is not the only agency within the US government with a stake in pharmaceutical issues. The Federal Trade Commission (FTC) has authority over general business practices in general. This of course includes the pharmacy business.

Federal Privacy Act

The Federal Privacy Act safeguards Americans against invasion of privacy through the misuse of records by federal agencies. Passed in 1974, the Privacy Act set up controls about what personal information can be collected, maintained, used and shared by agencies in the executive branch of the US government. This includes medical and pharmaceutical records.

Americans have the right to see their own records. They can also request changes to any records that are inaccurate, irrelevant, out of date or incomplete.

Americans are protected by The Privacy Act against unwarranted invasion of privacy that has resulted from the collection, maintenance, use, and disclosure of their personal information. If you feel your rights have been violated you can make a request under the Freedom of Information Act or the Federal Privacy Act.

Generic Substitution

What is a Generic Brand?

The pharmacist may discuss with your physician substituting a "no name" brand or an unbranded drug product in place of the drug brand specified by the physician.

The generic brand would have the same chemical makeup and the same dosage and drug form. It has been marketed by another company.

Generic Laws

Generic substitution laws vary from one state to another. Usually, a pharmacist cannot substitute a generic brand unless he can assure your physician that the generic drug contains the same active ingredient, in the same dosage and in the same form. It is critical that pharmacist use their professional judgment when substituting products to ensure patient safety and efficacy of the prescribed medicine.

For specific information about your state check out http://pharmacistsletter.therapeuticresearch.com/pl/ArticleDD.aspx?nidchk=1&cs=&s=PL&pt=2&segment=1186&dd=220901&AspxAutoDetectCookieSupport=1

Pharmacists and pharmacy technicians need to be aware of legal issues around substitution of a generic brand for the medication prescribed by the physician. The federal government regulates generic substitution. Pharmacists also need to be knowledgeable about state laws for their jurisdiction regarding generic substitution.

The following terms are relevant

Bioavialability: A test to determine if one drug has the same effect as the generic equivalent.

Bioequivalent drug products: Whether a generic drug is bioequivalent to the drug it is replacing is determined by: pharmacokinetic studies, pharmacodynamics investigations, comparative studies or vitro assessment.

Pharmaceutical equivalents are drug products that contain the same active ingredient(s), are of the same dosage and form, and are of identical strength as the prescribed medication.

Therapeutic equivalents: are drug products are considered to be pharmaceutical equivalents of the prescribed drug. If they are therapeutic equivalents they are expected to have the same healing effect and safety measures for patients when given under the the specified conditions on the label.

Orange Book: The Drug, Price and Competition Act states that the FDA must publish a list of approved drug products with therapeutic equivalence. The Orange Book's formal title is: *Orange Book: Approved Drug Products with Therapeutic Equivalence Evaluations.* The current book was good though April, 2015. The next edition is expected immediately. The products in the orange book list have been approved under section 505 of the Federal Food, Drug, and Cosmetic Act.

Professionals with Prescribing Authority

In an effort to improve health care in North America, more health professionals are being given the authority to prescribe and administer selected controlled substances. These healthcare professionals may include nurse practitioners, midwives, and podiatrists. They must be authorized to do so under state or provincial or territorial legislation.

These noted health professionals are currently able to prescribe other medications, such as antibiotics. However, in some states and provinces, they are currently not allowed to prescribe controlled substances including: codeine, fentanyl and diazepam. At this point the prescription o these is restricted to physicians, veterinarians and dentists under *Controlled Drugs and Substances Act. New Classes of Practitioners Regulations*—if passed—will allow nurse practitioners, midwives and podiatrists to prescribe and specific drugs containing controlled substances in the treatment of their patients.

Questions

Regulations and Technical Duties

1. A person must be a member of ………..in order for him to be a registered technician
   a. Institute of medicine
   b. College of pharmacists
   c. Food and drug administration
   d. Nurses society
2. The ………governs the licensing of pharmaceutical technicians
   a. Federal government
   b. State government
   c. Association of pharmacist
   d. College of pharmacist
3. The qualified pharmacy technician has no uniform specific certification until ……….
   a. 2016
   b. 2018
   c. 2020
   d. 2025
4. Which of the following body is responsible for governing the training of pharmacy technicians?
   a. Drug enforcement agents
   b. Food and drug administration
   c. College of pharmacists
   d. None of the above
5. Which of the following is a drawback of being unlicensed?
   a. It reduces employment opportunities
   b. It lowers remuneration bargaining power
   c. Higher responsibilities may not be assigned
   d. All of the above
6. When discussing with the customers, the pharmacist should ……..
   a. Warn them of any potential adverse reactions between the medication and food or beverages
   b. Make suggestions on when medication should be taken
   c. Listen to the patients concerns
   d. All of the above
7. Which of the following is a job of the pharmacy technician?
   a. Supervise the pharmacist
   b. Determining medication to be provided to patients
   c. Labeling bottles

d. Prescribing medications
8. Which of the following skills does a pharmacy technician need?
    a. Strong reporting skills
    b. Honesty
    c. Organizational skills
    d. All of the above
9. It is the responsibility of the pharmacist to …………
    a. Manage staff
    b. Maintain the pharmacy stock
    c. Ensure a clean pharmacy
    d. Issue bills
10. The pharmacy technician may……….
    a. Fill prescriptions
    b. Assess appropriateness of a prescription drug
    c. Calculate fees
    d. Interact with insurance companies
11. All of the following must be done by ONLY the pharmacist EXCEPT
    a. Dialogue with medical professionals regarding potential adverse effects of prescribed drugs
    b. Record charges
    c. File a claim
    d. Counsel patients on clinical issues
12. Prescriptions can be received …………
    a. In person
    b. Via internet
    c. Via fax
    d. All of the above
13. In order to avoid confusion, the prescription department should …………
    a. Have the same work station for every staff
    b. One window for both receiving and dispensing of drugs
    c. Have a data entry area
    d. Have one shelf for bottles and files
14. Which of the following is done first when there is an order?
    a. Check patients file for allergies
    b. Orders are signed
    c. Refill prescriptions
    d. Record prescriptions
15. To achieve maximum efficiency of the pharmacy's prescription department…………
    a. There should not be division of labor
    b. Personnel should not get into each others way
    c. A tiny space should be used
    d. All of the above
16. To ensure adequate security which of the following should be done

a. An alarm system should be installed
b. There should be adequate backup in case of power outage
c. Keys should be numbered
d. All of the above

17. Which of the following should be done to ensure the safety of keys?
    a. Ensure keys are duplicated
    b. Only Opening procedures should be in place
    c. Keys are should be numbered
    d. All of the above

18. Closed circuit TV should be installed ………..
    a. In the parking lot
    b. Lunch room
    c. In the restroom
    d. None of the above

19. Camera should be audited ………
    a. Every six months
    b. Every week
    c. Every year
    d. Every 2 years

20. In the event of burglary, staff should ……..
    a. Call the police
    b. Fight with the burglars
    c. Protect the drug inventory aggressively
    d. All of the above

21. Accurate inventory control is important because ……….
    a. The health of others is at stake
    b. The company's reputation is at stake
    c. The company's profit is at stake
    d. The company's cost will decrease

22. Good inventory control ensures that …………
    a. There is minimum overstocking
    b. Patients get their prescription in a timely manner
    c. There is a knowledge of what is in stock at any time
    d. All of the above

23. Inventory control in a pharmacy is difficult because ………
    a. Medications may change
    b. Staff may change
    c. Prices of products may increase
    d. Doctors may change

24. Pharmacies are expected to do which of the following?
    a. Keep a wide range of stock
    b. Make bulk purchase

c. Turn over inventory without extra cost
d. All of the above

25. .... Method of inventory control allots fund in a specific timeframe to buy pharmaceutical inventory
    a. Short list method
    b. Minimum and maximum method
    c. Open-to-buy budget
    d. Stock card method

26. The ....method singles of products in low stock and flags them for the pharmaceutical technician to replace
    a. Short list method
    b. Stock card method
    c. Minimum and maximum method
    d. Open-to-buy budget

27. The minimum and maximum method ....
    a. Traces the items that are about to expire
    b. Discovers how much of the item to order and the best time financially to order
    c. Traces when items are purchased
    d. Flags low stock items

28. The .... Traces when items are purchased by using notations on cards or e-cards
    a. Notation cards
    b. Stock cards
    c. Kardex
    d. Short list cards

29. Dispensing errors account for over .... Of medication mistakes
    a. 2%
    b. 5%
    c. 10%
    d. 20%

30. Dispensing error can result in ....
    a. Potential loss of life
    b. Increased healthcare cost
    c. Law suit
    d. All of the above

31. Dispensing error can be avoided if ....
    a. Stock cards are used
    b. Inventory is stored in marked and consistent locations
    c. Staffs are changed regularly
    d. Prescriptions are not changed

32. Which of the following increases dispensing errors?
    a. Good lighting
    b. Optimum temperature

c. Clustered counter space
d. All of the above

33. When dispensing drugs ………
    a. Label after all prescriptions have been dispensed
    b. Deal with one medication at a time
    c. Dispense and label immediately
    d. All of the above

34. To avoid mix up …………
    a. Store medications that look alike in different storage area
    b. Labels should be facing front
    c. Medications should be properly organized
    d. All of the above

35. Expired products should be ……….
    a. Sold at half price
    b. Sold at full price
    c. Discarded
    d. Burnt

36. Most injectable epinephrine products expires ……after the product arrives for stocking on the shelves
    a. 6 months
    b. 10 months
    c. 18 months
    d. 36 months

37. Which of the following is true?
    a. It is dangerous to use out of date drugs
    b. It is unethical to sell out of date drugs
    c. It is illegal to sell out of date drugs
    d. All of the above

38. Which of the following makes the manufacturers expiry date no longer valid?
    a. Transferring drugs to another container
    b. Changing the shelf location of the drug
    c. Selling the drug
    d. All of the above

39. The stability of a medication may be compromised if it is introduced to …………
    a. Heat
    b. A new shelf
    c. A new packaging
    d. Another pharmacy

40. Which of the following should be considered before disposing expired drugs?
    a. Regulations regarding safe disposal in the jurisdiction
    b. The form of the medication
    c. Whether it can be returned to the manufacturers

d. All of the above
41. Which of the following should be recorded when discarding drugs?
    a. The quantity
    b. The location of disposal
    c. How it was disposed
    d. All of the above
42. When disposing drugs ....
    a. It must be witnessed by a government official
    b. The disposal must be captured on CCTV
    c. A licensed pharmacist must be present
    d. It must be done within the pharmacy
43. Safeguarding controlled substances is a concern for ....
    a. Manufacturers
    b. Distributors
    c. Pharmacies
    d. All of the above
44. ....specifies the handling of controlled substances
    a. State law
    b. Federal law
    c. Pharmacy policy
    d. Pharmacy procedure
45. Which of the following regulates storage and sales of controlled substances?
    a. Controlled Drugs and Substances Act
    b. Narcotics Drug Act
    c. Food and Narcotics Control regulations
    d. All of the above
46. Controlled substances in North America must have ....
    a. 10 digit code
    b. 8 digit DIN numerical code
    c. 4 digit control code
    d. 76 digit DIN numerical code
47. Controlled substances may be diverted through ....
    a. Illegal sale
    b. Employee theft
    c. Robbery
    d. All of the above
48. To prevent diversion employees..........
    a. Should be rotated
    b. Should be screened
    c. Should be well paid
    d. Should be given pay rise often
49. Which of the following should be done before employees are hired?

    a. Evaluate personal references
    b. Carry out background checks
    c. Verify previous place of employment
    d. All of the above
50. To ensure the safety of controlled substances …………..
    a. Controlled substances are should be secured
    b. Many employees should be assigned to that unit to ensure delegation of duties
    c. Employees working there should wear their ID all the time
    d. A register should be opened to monitor movement
51. Which of the following must be considered when securing controlled substances?
    a. The location of the pharmacy
    b. The form of controlled substances
    c. The activities involved in handling controlled substances
    d. All of the above
52. To ensure maximum security of controlled substances, ……..
    a. The alarm system should be adequately supervised
    b. Entrance to controlled substance area should be monitored
    c. Public access to the building should be supervised and controlled
    d. All of the above
53. Drugs and medication considered controlled substances are divided into ………schedules
    a. 3
    b. 4
    c. 5
    d. 6
54. The designation of the schedule is based on which of the following criteria?
    a. Whether it has an approved medical use in the United State
    b. The likelihood of the substance causing dependence
    c. The abuse potential of the substance
    d. All of the above
55. Which of the following is true about substances in schedule I
    a. There is no currently accepted medical use
    b. It is safe for medical use
    c. It has medical use
    d. All of the above
56. Which of the following is an example of substances in schedule I
    a. Percocet
    b. Peyote
    c. Methadone
    d. Demerol
57. Substances in schedule ……… lack accepted safety for medical use
    a. I
    b. II

c. III
d. IV

58. Which of the following is an example of drugs in schedule II
    a. Heroin
    b. Opium
    c. Peyote
    d. Lysergic acid diethylamide
59. Which of the following is true about schedule III?
    a. It has a high potential for abuse
    b. It is not accepted for medical use
    c. It may lead to moderate physical dependence
    d. All of the above
60. Which of the following is categorized under schedule III
    a. Ketamine
    b. Morphine
    c. Oxycodone
    d. Peyote
61. Which of the following is true about substances in schedule IV?
    a. It has potential of being abused
    b. It is not safe for medical use
    c. It has less potential for abuse
    d. There is tendency for high psychological dependence
62. Which of the following substances is categorized under schedule IV?
    a. Ketamine
    b. Soma
    c. Codeine
    d. Demerol
63. Substances in schedule .... have the lowest potential for abuse
    a. V
    b. IV
    c. III
    d. I
64. All of the following are examples of substances in schedule V EXCEPT
    a. Ezogabine
    b. Xanax
    c. Robitussin AC
    d. Phenergan with codeine
65. Which of the following must be included on the prescription?
    a. Dosage form
    b. Strength
    c. Name of medication
    d. All of the above

66. The prescription must be signed by the ....
    a. Nurse
    b. Secretary
    c. Practitioner
    d. Technician
67. Which of the following is true for controlled substances?
    a. Electronic prescriptions are allowed on any software
    b. All pharmacies are permitted to receive electronic prescriptions
    c. Only DEA-registered pharmacies are permitted to archive electronic prescription
    d. All of the above
68. A doctor may issue multiple prescriptions for up to a ....supply of schedule II controlled substances
    a. Thirty day
    b. Forty-five day
    c. Ninety day
    d. One hundred day
69. Which of the following conditions must exist before a doctor can issue multiple prescriptions of a schedule II controlled substance?
    a. Each prescription must be on a separate prescription blank
    b. Each prescription is for a medically legitimate purpose
    c. It must be legal under the state law
    d. All of the above
70. Which of the following is true?
    a. Schedule III may be refilled if a refill note was included on the prescription
    b. Schedule II may be refilled in the pharmacy
    c. Schedule II may be refilled if a refill note was included
    d. All of the above
71. Schedule III controlled substances may be refilled up to ....within six months
    a. Two times
    b. Five times
    c. Six times
    d. Seven times
72. In the case of partial filling, ...
    a. The pharmacist must inform the DEA
    b. The pharmacist must make note of the quantity supplied
    c. The pharmacist must sign a declaration form
    d. All of the above
73. All of the following should be done after giving a partial prescription EXCEPT?
    a. The remainder may be dispensed within one week
    b. If remainder can't be dispensed within 3 weeks the issuing doctor must be notified
    c. The remaining may be dispensed within 72 hours
    d. A new prescription will be issued to replace the partially filled one after 72 hours

74. Drugs classified under schedule .... of the uniform controlled substances act can be dispensed without a prescription
    a. II
    b. III
    c. V
    d. IV
75. Schedule V controlled substances can be sold under which of the following guidelines?
    a. The product should be sold only in a pharmacy
    b. It should be sold to patients over 18 years
    c. The purchaser's name and address should be verified
    d. It can be displayed in an accessible location
76. Which of the following guidelines should be adhered to?
    a. The name of the pharmacy selling should be affixed to the bottle
    b. The purchaser should be provided with a copy of subsection 3 and 4 of schedule V drugs
    c. There should be a schedule V register book in every pharmacy
    d. All of the above
77. Which of the following must be written on the top of each page of the schedule V register?
    a. I have not obtained any schedule V preparations within the last 3 days
    b. I am not a drug addict
    c. This is my true name and address
    d. I thereby solemnly swear
78. Which of the following should be recorded in the schedule V register when a sale is made without doctor's prescription?
    a. Date of sale
    b. Name and quantity of controlled substance
    c. Proof of identification
    d. All of the above
79. The register must ....
    a. Be bound
    b. Be colored
    c. Be 11 by 13 inches
    d. Be black
80. The duplicate pages of the schedule V register must be mailed to the ....at the end of each month
    a. Drug Enforcement Agency
    b. Food and drug administration
    c. Pharmacy board
    d. Doctor
81. The controlled substances Act is a ....policy
    a. State
    b. Federal
    c. Municipal

d. Pharmacy
82. The Controlled Substances Act regulates the …………..of all substances deemed to be controlled
   a. Manufacture
   b. Importing
   c. Possession
   d. All of the above
83. The Drug Enforcement Administration and the ……….decides what substances should be added, removed or moved from each of the schedules
   a. Federal Bureau of Investigators
   b. Food and Drug Administration
   c. Members of college of Pharmacy
   d. Doctors Association
84. Which of the following is true about DEA numbers?
   a. They are used to track controlled substances
   b. A person without DEA number may issue prescriptions only during emergencies
   c. It comprises of 3 letters
   d. It is made up of four numbers
85. All of the following can be assigned DEA numbers EXCEPT
   a. Doctor
   b. Veterinarian
   c. Pharmacy technician
   d. Dentist
86. In the United States, food, drugs cosmetics and medical devices are regulated by the …………
   a. Food and Drug Administration
   b. National Institutes of Health
   c. Healthcare Financing Administration
   d. Centers for Disease Control and Prevention
87. Which of the following is a function of the FDA?
   a. They inspect manufacturing facilities
   b. They test products
   c. They monitor research
   d. All of the above
88. The ……….has authority over general business practices
   a. The Center for Food Safety and Applied Nutrition
   b. The Federal Trade Commission
   c. Healthcare Financing Administration
   d. National Institutes of Health
89. All of the following are components of the FDA EXCEPT
   a. Center for Disease Control and Prevention
   b. The Center for Drug Evaluation and Research
   c. The Center for Veterinary Medicine
   d. National Center for Toxicological Research

90. Most prescription drugs are evaluated by the ....
    a. Center for Drug Assessment and Evaluation
    b. The center for Food Safety and Applied Nutrition
    c. Center for Drug Evaluation and Research
    d. The National Center for Research and Assessment
91. The Federal Privacy Act ensures ....
    a. Records are not misused
    b. Drugs can be prescribed in privacy
    c. Prescriptions can be sent secretly
    d. All of the above
92. Americans have which of the following rights?
    a. Right to see their own records
    b. Right to request changes to inaccurate records
    c. Right to request changes to incomplete records
    d. All of the above
93. Which of the following is true about generic drugs?
    a. It is branded
    b. It has the same chemical makeup as the specified drug
    c. It is marketed by the same company
    d. All of the above
94. Substitution can occur if the drug has the same ....
    a. Active ingredient
    b. Color
    c. Packaging
    d. Shape
95. The .... can substitute drugs.
    a. Pharmacist
    b. Nurse
    c. Pharmacy technician
    d. Nursing assistant
96. .... is a test to determine if one drug has the same effect as the generic equivalent
    a. Toxicology test
    b. Bioavailability test
    c. Acidity test
    d. Biostability test
97. Whether a generic drug is bioequivalent to the drug it is replacing is determined by ....
    a. Pharmacokinetics studies
    b. Pharmacotherapeutics investigation
    c. Pharmacology review
    d. All of the above
98. Which of the following is true about a pharmaceutical equivalent?
    a. The price is the same as the prescribed drug

b. The dosage and form is the same as the prescribed drug
   c. The packaging is the same as the prescribed drug
   d. All of the above
99. Therapeutic equivalents are expected to have the same ....
   a. Healing effect
   b. Inactive ingredient
   c. Quantity
   d. Dosage
100.   Currently ....can prescribe diazepam
   a. Nurse practitioners
   b. Midwives
   c. Dentists
   d. Podiatrists

Answers

1. B
2. B
3. C
4. D
5. D
6. D
7. C
8. D
9. A
10. C
11. B
12. D
13. C
14. A
15. B
16. D
17. C
18. A
19. B
20. A
21. A
22. D
23. A
24. D
25. C
26. A
27. B
28. B
29. D
30. D
31. B
32. C
33. C
34. D
35. C
36. C
37. D
38. A
39. A
40. D
41. D
42. C

43. D
44. B
45. A
46. B
47. D
48. B
49. D
50. A
51. D
52. D
53. C
54. D
55. A
56. B
57. A
58. B
59. C
60. A
61. C
62. B
63. A
64. B
65. D
66. C
67. C
68. C
69. D
70. A
71. B
72. B
73. A
74. C
75. C
76. D
77. C
78. D
79. A
80. C
81. B
82. D
83. B
84. A
85. C
86. A
87. D
88. B
89. A
90. C

91. A
92. D
93. C
94. A
95. A
96. B
97. A
98. B
99. A
100. C

www.ingramcontent.com/pod-product-compliance
Lightning Source LLC
Chambersburg PA
CBHW081800170526
45167CB00008B/3267